KEVIN KENDALL

# 21 Rules for Digestive Health

# Contents

# Introduction

"You are what you eat."

This familiar saying underscores the importance of diet in achieving good health. Indeed, our physical bodies are largely composed of what we consume. However, understanding what constitutes a healthy diet is more complex than following broad guidelines like the food pyramid.

The food pyramid, rooted more in economic considerations than nutrition, suggests a diet dominated by fruits, vegetables, and grains, with minimal meat and fats. Despite this model, obesity and chronic disease rates continue to rise, indicating that the advice is perhaps not the pinnacle of human achievement.

My journey with Crohn's Disease has taught me this first-hand. After numerous failed attempts to control my condition with medication and surgery, I realised that the treatments were harming me more than helping. Controlling the disease through diet became my only option. Conventional wisdom about healthy eating didn't work for me; in fact, it exacerbated my symptoms. Through trial and error, I discovered that much of the accepted advice was perpetuating my illness.

Digestive health is highly individual—what works for one person may not work for another. This uniqueness complicates the identification of dietary causes of digestive diseases.

Another complication is related to the effect of many different influencing factors. While science is often more than happy to classify individual chemicals as safe for consumption, it is somewhat more reticent to investigate the impact of repeated exposure to multiple substances. This raises questions about the long-term effects of these cumulative interactions on human health.

Some of my rules are tailored to managing inflammation and ulceration, while others are probably more universally beneficial. One key observation is that the foods causing damage to the gut may not immediately cause noticeable symptoms. The bowel lacks pain receptors, so initial damage often goes unnoticed until secondary symptoms arise.

My rules aren't about preaching perfection but finding a balance. I don't adhere to them entirely, but applying them most of the time has greatly improved my health. I find it helps to picture good and bad foods balancing on a set of scales - as long as the scales are tipping towards the positive side then all is good.

Much of the problem lies with processed foods, now called ultra-processed foods. Despite the new terminology, these are the same products that have long been problematic.

You might find some or all of these rules helpful. Adopting even a few could make a significant difference. Whether you're dealing with a specific condition or simply seeking better health, my guidelines can offer a new perspective and practical solutions.

I have deliberately provided references to relatively straightforward supporting evidence throughout this book. The reason for doing so is that I have built these rules from direct experience rather than from an academic perspective. The supporting evidence is just that – 'supporting' being the important part. If I do all of, or at least most of, the following, then I can defy medical expectations. I don't need scientific studies to confirm my relative good health.

So, rather than rambling on about nothing, I'll get straight to my rules. They are not in any specific order of importance, so you can start at the start or dive in wherever you feel like.

# 1

# Rule 1: Don't Eat Maltodextrin

Maltodextrin refers to a range of molecules, not just one. They are all white powders and are water-soluble.

There is digestible maltodextrin. It is a simple chain of glucose molecules, between 3 and 17 molecules long. I don't know why the lower and upper limits are defined as such, but that is the case according to Wikipedia. Since it isn't particularly relevant to what I want to discuss I'll take their word for it (although other sources state the upper chain length to be 20).

The starting point of digestible maltodextrin is a starch such as corn, wheat, or potato. Starch is the term used to describe long chains of glucose molecules. A process called hydrolysis is applied to the starch. In English, water, acids, enzymes, and heat break each long starch molecule into multiple smaller chains. The extent of hydrolysis can be controlled, meaning the properties of the resulting maltodextrin can be adjusted, allowing for differences in sweetness, texture, and viscosity (viscosity refers to the thickness of a liquid).

There is also digestion-resistant maltodextrin, but that is not what I'm focusing on here. It appears on food labels as soluble fibre (fiber if you are American), resistant dextrin, or just dextrin.

## Why Use It?

Digestible maltodextrin was first produced as a food additive in the late 1960s and early 1970s. Since then, it has found its way into a wide range of processed foods and drinks. It is used as a bulking agent and a sugar substitute, as well as for texture and flavour enhancement. It can be found in baby food, sports supplements, and of note for what I am writing about, medical supplements. It also finds its way into table sauces, gravy and stock mixes, and the coatings on various snack foods.

## What's The Problem?

The timeline I just mentioned is interesting as it correlates nicely with the modern explosion of inflammatory bowel disease. I'll not focus on this because correlation doesn't necessarily prove causation.

Maltodextrin is classed as a complex carbohydrate. The food industry uses it to lower the apparent sugar content in manufactured products. However, it has a glycemic index ranging from 85 to 105 depending on the specific maltodextrin, close to or even above pure glucose (100). Regular sugar (sucrose) has a glycemic index of around 65.

This means maltodextrin produces a more pronounced blood sugar spike than sugar and even glucose in some cases. So if sugar causes diabetes, then maltodextrin is even worse. Yet manufacturers get to list it as a complex carbohydrate, implying health benefits over sugar. They can even boast about how low in sugar their products are, even though basic sugar wouldn't be as bad.

As with the correlation to the increased prevalence of IBD, while this is something worth taking note of, it isn't the reason I avoid it.

I had the worst version of Crohn's Disease for many years. One of the effects of the disease is weight loss, due to not being able to eat.

Medicine addresses this issue by prescribing high-calorie nutritional supplements to patients. These are full of vitamins and minerals, and the calorie content is usually added via maltodextrin.

The increased nutrition should, in principle, address the issues of malnutrition that come with the disease, but I always found my health would get worse when I was taking these supplements. Long before I had any additional evidence, I had identified maltodextrin as having a negative effect, through simple observation of my condition.

My doctors dismissed these concerns whenever I brought them up.

It took a long time before I decided to look for some science that might confirm my suspicions...

One paper, **Maltodextrin, Modern Stressor of the Intestinal Environment**, starts with the following introduction...

> *A critically important new study by Laudisi et al shows that consumption of the food additive maltodextrin, incorporated into many processed foods, leads to the promotion of intestinal inflammation. These findings suggest that this broadly used food additive could be a risk factor for chronic inflammatory diseases.*

That quote seems self-explanatory.

Another, **Maltodextrin Consumption Impairs the Intestinal Mucus Barrier and Accelerates Colitis Through Direct Actions on the Epithelium**, provides this quote...

> *In this study, we investigated two common food additives, MDX and CMC, using a colitis-prone mouse model driven by both host genetics and microbes, allowing us to investigate the integration of several risk factors on chronic disease activity. Both MDX and*

*CMC accelerated the onset and severity of intestinal and systemic inflammation, altered the microbiome profile and function, and decreased intestinal mucus production.*

In that quote, MDX refers to maltodextrin. CMC is carboxymethyl cellulose (a cellulose gum derived from plant fibres)

Yet another study says it all in the title, **Crohn's Disease-Associated Adherent-Invasive *Escherichia coli* Adhesion Is Enhanced by Exposure to the Ubiquitous Dietary Polysaccharide Maltodextrin**

There's no reason to pull quotes from that one to help explain it here.

## Final Points

There is some ambiguity as to why a short chain of glucose molecules can have such a detrimental effect, as in theory, it is quickly broken down to glucose in the digestive tract, so it shouldn't pose such a problem.

One theory is that the body must use excessive amounts of specific digestive enzymes to break the maltodextrin molecules down. The supply of these enzymes becomes depleted, leaving whole molecules undigested, which provides a food source for unwanted forms of bacteria. While this may be the case, my reasoning tends towards the effect of undigested bits of food on the digestive lining itself.

That is why I avoid maltodextrin.

# Further Reading

**Maltodextrin - Wikipedia**

*https://en.wikipedia.org/wiki/Maltodextrin*

**Maltodextrin, Modern Stressor of the Intestinal Environment**

*https://www.ncbi.nlm.nih.gov/pmc/articles/PMC6409436/*

**Maltodextrin Consumption Impairs the Intestinal Mucus Barrier and Accelerates Colitis Through Direct Actions on the Epithelium**

*https://www.ncbi.nlm.nih.gov/pmc/articles/PMC8963984/*

**Crohn's Disease-Associated Adherent-Invasive Escherichia coli Adhesion Is Enhanced by Exposure to the Ubiquitous Dietary Polysaccharide Maltodextrin**

*https://www.ncbi.nlm.nih.gov/pmc/articles/PMC3520894/*

2

# Rule 2: Don't Eat Soap

Up until recently, I hadn't thought much about the role of, and the extent of, emulsifiers in food, and also hadn't considered the potential for negative health consequences.

Many foods include water and oil in the ingredients, and these don't mix well.

An emulsifier solves this problem. It is a molecule with dual properties. One part will attract water, and the other will attract oil, resulting in mixtures where the water and oil are happy to exist in the same space.

If you have ever read a list of ingredients and wondered what mono and diglycerides of fatty acids are, they are emulsifiers. They are made by reacting edible oils with glycerol. This involves heat and a catalyst such as sodium hydroxide (caustic soda) or potassium hydroxide (lye).

Lecithins are emulsifiers. They are extracted from seed oils, such as soybean, sunflower, or rapeseed. The chemicals used to extract lecithin from an oil include hexane, benzene, petroleum ether, and acetone — all nice and wholesome.

Diphosphates are used as emulsifiers. In general terms, these are produced by reacting phosphoric acid with a hydroxide (caustic soda or lye)

Xanthan gum and pectin are also used as emulsifiers. Xanthan gum is made by fermenting sugar with a bacteria called Xanthomonas Campestris. Various other gums have emulsifying properties (Acacia, Arabic, Guar). Pectin is made from fruit.

This is by no means the full set of emulsifiers found in foods. Other, more exotic chemicals include Carrageenan, Carboxymethyl Cellulose (CMC), Microcrystalline Cellulose, Maltodextrin, and Polysorbate-80, to name but a few.

Many foods will have more than one emulsifier listed in the ingredients.

There is a crossover between ingredients — ones that are used for emulsifying and ones that are used as thickening or stabilising agents. In all, there are over 100 different food additives that can fulfil the role of an emulsifier.

## Why Use It?

If the oil and water in a food separate from one another, then that food stops being nice and edible and becomes spoiled. The longer a food sits for, the more likelihood there is of this.

Such a situation isn't good for business. After surviving manufacturing processes and long distribution chains, food sits on supermarket shelves for varying amounts of time, then once purchased, it is placed in cupboards and fridges until eaten. The last thing a consumer wants is to buy food, only to discover it is off by the time they eat it.

Emulsifiers extend the shelf life of products, making it possible for the processed food industry to exist.

Other properties include the likes of making bread softer and ice cream smoother.

In the UK, 51% of all food contains at least one emulsifier. They are in 95% of commercially produced bakery products, 81% of milk-based drinks, 81% of manufactured desserts, and 77% of confectionery items.

All in all, that's a lot of food containing emulsifiers.

Centralised food production and distribution brings many conveniences for consumers, and opens up endless opportunities for large-scale manufacturing.

Classed as safe by various food standards agencies, emulsifiers are very well represented in foods that come in a packet with an ingredient list. They are one of those under-the-radar kinds of ingredients, ones that don't catch your attention unless you are specifically looking.

## What's the Problem?

To recap the basic properties of an emulsifier, it will bind to both water and fat.

In terms of digestion, the body's first line of defence is a mucous membrane that coats the cells of the digestive system. This helps stop potential irritants from making contact with and causing damage to actual cells. Mucous is 95% water. The other 5% is lipids (fatty substances), electrolytes, and proteins.

An emulsifier will attract water and fats, both found in mucous — so it can dissolve parts of that mucous. In simpler terms, it can strip away the protective digestive lining.

If you want some science to back up my general idea that emulsifiers are bad, then **Emulsifiers Make Food Appetizing yet Bring Health Dangers**, an article on WebMD is a good starting point. Here's a quote from the introduction...

*Evidence links emulsifiers with upset gut microbiome, inflamma-tion, and several conditions, from heart attacks to breast cancer.*

Another paper, **Food additives: Assessing the impact of exposure to permitted emulsifiers on bowel and metabolic health — introducing the FADiets study**, has the following quote in the opening paragraph...

*This raises the possibility that dietary emulsifiers might be factors in conditions such as coronary artery disease, type 2 diabetes and Crohn's disease.*

Yet another, **Food Additive Emulsifiers and Their Impact on Gut Microbiome, Permeability, and Inflammation: Mechanistic Insights in Inflammatory Bowel Disease**, has the following in the opening few sentences...

*There is growing evidence that aspects of a 'Western diet' increase the risk of developing IBD. More recently, evidence implicating dietary emulsifiers has accumulated, with ecological studies show-ing a positive correlation between inflammatory bowel disease and emulsifier consumption.*

## Final Points

Production of some of the most common emulsifiers is similar to soaps and detergents, which are also made by reacting fats or oils with hydroxides. The action of detergents is also very similar — they are even described as 'having an emulsifying effect'.

I know I shouldn't eat soap. That is why I avoid emulsifiers.

# Further Reading

**Emulsifiers in ultra-processed foods in the United Kingdom food supply**

*https://www.researchgate.net/publication/374092790_Emulsifiers_in_ultra-processed_foods_in_the_United_Kingdom_food_supply*

**Emulsifiers Make Food Appetizing yet Bring Health Dangers**
*https://www.webmd.com/diet/news/20240412/emulsifiers-in-food-may-bring-health-dangers*

**Food additives: Assessing the impact of exposure to permitted emulsifiers on bowel and metabolic health – introducing the FADiets study**

*https://www.ncbi.nlm.nih.gov/pmc/articles/PMC6899614/*

**Food Additive Emulsifiers and Their Impact on Gut Microbiome, Permeability, and Inflammation: Mechanistic Insights in Inflammatory Bowel Disease**

*https://pubmed.ncbi.nlm.nih.gov/33336247/*

# 3

# Rule 3: Don't Eat Sawdust

You might be wondering why I chose to use the word 'sawdust' in the title of this chapter. I promise it wasn't a clickbait type of decision. There is good reason to describe **microcrystalline cellulose** this way.

Rather than me explaining, here's a quote from Wikipedia…

> *Microcrystalline cellulose (MCC) is a term for refined wood pulp and is used as a texturizer, an anti-caking agent, a fat substitute, an emulsifier, an extender, and a bulking agent in food production*

As the name implies, wood pulp starts as wood or sawdust. This is turned into microcrystalline cellulose via a variety of industrial processes. So, in an almost literal sense, it is wood.

The resulting product consists of microscopically small crystals. The size of the crystals has a lot of relevance concerning the reasons I avoid it. In terms of what it looks like in its raw form, it is a fine white powder.

## Why Use It?

Microcrystalline cellulose has a lot of uses in processed food.

It is used as a texturiser, meaning it enhances the texture of products. It is also an anti-caking agent, so will stop powders from clumping together. It can be used as a fat substitute in low-fat products. It has emulsifying properties, so helps mix water and oil. It is also a bulking agent, meaning it can add volume to a food product without adding calories.

It is used extensively in the pharmaceutical and nutritional supplement industries, as the base ingredient of tablets.

It is used in cosmetics, where one of its functions is to act as an abrasive.

It is classed as being inert. This implies it does not affect the digestive system.

It is even sold as a weight loss supplement. If you fill up on microcrystalline cellulose, you won't feel as hungry for real food.

## What's the Problem?

If I were to believe the pronouncements of food standards and safety organisations and the medical industry, then there is no problem. For the vast majority of the population, this probably is the case.

However, if you have inflammation in your digestive system, then there is every chance it is having a very different effect.

Think of the digestive system as being a sieve. This, quite literally, is what it is. The function of the bowel is to let nutrients through to the bloodstream and keep bigger molecules out. Even though the crystals of microcrystalline cellulose are microscopic, they still fall into the category of bigger molecules. The only ones that should get through the digestive barrier are even smaller than this.

However, a damaged bowel has ulcers and inflammation in places where there should be a tightly meshed cellular structure. The default way of thinking about inflammatory bowel disease suggests that absorption of nutrients is impaired because of this. But if you flip your thinking around, it is equally, if not more valid to assume that damaged areas will be letting a lot more through than they should.

Thinking about a kitchen sieve is a good way of picturing this. When the sieve is fully intact, it will do what it is supposed to and will sift out any lumps in whatever is being sieved, only letting the fine particles through. If you cut some holes in the sieve, it will allow the big lumps through with the finer particles.

Ulcers are the biological equivalent of cutting holes in the sieve.

So, it is fair to assume that if you have digestive inflammation, which tends to go hand in hand with ulceration, particles that should be kept out of the bloodstream are much more likely to get through. This will trigger an inflammatory response, as the body is tasked with containing and eliminating the particles. Hence the incurable nature of inflammatory bowel disease.

Microcrystalline cellulose ticks all of the boxes for such a scenario. It is perfectly safe for most, but if my hypothesis is anywhere near correct, it is going to cause even more damage in people with pre-existing digestive damage. I've already mentioned its use as an abrasive in cosmetics.

## Final Points

Remember also, that it is used as the base for the tablets doctors are eager to prescribe.

Where possible and relevant, I'm providing links to scientific papers backing up my claims for this series of rules about digestive health. Even though I am convinced microcrystalline cellulose is not good, and direct evidence backs up my position, the science errs towards the opposite viewpoint, stating (rather ambiguously) that it can help in diseases such as Crohn's and Colitis. The science also states that Crohn's is incurable.

I'd argue otherwise. That is why I don't eat sawdust.


## Further Reading


**Wikipedia: Microcrystalline Cellulose**

*https://en.wikipedia.org/wiki/Microcrystalline_cellulose*

4

# Rule 4: Don't Eat Coal Tar Derivatives

Coal Tar is made by heating coal, in the absence of oxygen, to temperatures ranging from 900 to 1200 degrees Celsius. It is good for treating psoriasis and dandruff but was listed as a known carcinogen in 1980. While it might be good at treating a flaky scalp, it isn't something most of us would consider eating.

Anthranilic acid is one of the main components of coal tar, although it can also be synthesised, so I'll admit I'm taking a bit of a liberty with the title of this chapter. However, in the context of the history of what I'm talking about, coal tar was originally the raw material.

Anthranilic acid, when reacted with nitrous acid, sulphur dioxide, chlorine, and ammonia, becomes the artificial sweetener known as **saccharin**.

## Why Use It?

Saccharin was the original fully artificial sweetener, first discovered in 1879. It first gained popularity during the First World War due to sugar shortages. It then gained considerably more popularity in the 1960s and

1970s as an answer to obesity.

There were attempts to ban it completely when it was alleged to cause bladder cancer in rats.

Rather than being banned outright in the USA, it carried a health warning until the year 2000, when the warning was dropped because new research concluded humans didn't suffer the same effects as rats.

This leads one to wonder, that if this is the case, why are rats used to prove the safety and effectiveness of anything?

Canada did ban it completely. However, since rats yielded the wrong answer regarding the safety of saccharin, the Canadians have rolled back their decision and allowed the chemical to be used as a tabletop sweetener. They are also looking into allowing broader use across the processed food industry.

These days it is great according to food standards agencies. Call me conspiratorial if you wish, but I'd rather not take the risk, in a 'just in case' kind of way.

Regarding inflammatory bowel disease, at least one study offers evidence to suggest saccharin inhibits colitis. This research was done with mice. It's a good job they chose mice rather than rats. If it had been a study on rats, the evidence would have been meaningless since humans and rats don't appear to exhibit the same effects when given chemicals (although that might only be the case when health warnings are eating into corporate profits).

## What's The Problem?

There is evidence to suggest that saccharin reduces biodiversity in the gut. The subject of digestive bacteria opens up a world of circular reasoning, going beyond the scope of what I am covering here. My stance on this subject tends towards bacteria being the result of underlying health rather than the cause (this will crop up in a few other places in these rules).

Scientific literature is ambiguous. The NIH article, **Overall Evaluations of Carcinogenicity: An Updating of IARC Monographs Volumes 1 to 42**, says the evidence for carcinogenicity in humans is 'inadequate', whereas the evidence for carcinogenicity in animals is 'sufficient'.

That article is based on lots of studies, and to be fair, the evidence of bladder cancer in rodents was produced by injecting saccharin directly into their bladders, so there aren't going to be any human studies to back up the findings, due to the ethics of doing such a thing.

An argument that is repeated, time and time again for artificial ingredients is the one that we do not consume enough of any given substance for it to have toxic effects. I'd argue that any amount of poison is too much, rather than trying to claim it is perfectly safe below some arbitrary threshold.

There is also evidence to suggest saccharin causes a list of other health problems. Here's a quote from **Long-Term Saccharin Consumption and Increased Risk of Obesity, Diabetes, Hepatic Dysfunction, and Renal Impairment in Rats**...

> *The results obtained in the present study suggest that long-term saccharin consumption increases the risk of obesity and diabetes, as well as liver and renal impairment. The results also suggest an increased risk of brain carcinogenesis.*

This was a study on rats so feel free to take whatever message you want from that, given that the rat study linking saccharin to bladder cancer turned out to be irrelevant to humans.

## Final Points

As is often the case with scientific studies, the research on saccharin offers little concrete evidence either way. However, it does illustrate the limits of science. As complexity increases, understanding often does the opposite.

I have learned to err towards caution in situations like this.

I've never been anywhere close to being overweight, so do not need to limit my calorie intake. As such, I'm not well-placed to judge its value in terms of weight loss.

The best argument that can be put forward regarding the effects of saccharin on health is that it isn't toxic enough to be of concern, and that is not a very strong argument.

However, it is absorbed by the body, so the body is tasked with eliminating it. It doesn't provide any nutritional value, so in terms of net value, it is a drain on resources.

The human body does not recognise saccharin as having any biological use whatsoever. Rather than someone such as myself having to prove it is bad for health, I'd argue the responsibility lies with manufacturers to show that it isn't. In more than a century, they haven't managed to.

That is why I don't eat saccharin.

# Further Reading

**Wikipedia – Saccharin**

*https://en.wikipedia.org/wiki/Saccharin*

**Overall Evaluations of Carcinogenicity: An Updating of IARC Mono-graphs Volumes 1 to 42**

*https://www.ncbi.nlm.nih.gov/books/NBK533616/*

**Saccharin Supplementation Inhibits Bacterial Growth and Reduces Experimental Colitis in Mice**

*https://www.ncbi.nlm.nih.gov/pmc/articles/PMC7230785/*

**Long-Term Saccharin Consumption and Increased Risk of Obesity, Diabetes, Hepatic Dysfunction, and Renal Impairment in Rats**

*https://www.ncbi.nlm.nih.gov/pmc/articles/PMC6843803/*

5

# Rule 5: Don't Eat Cyanide

Everyone has heard of cyanide, and everyone knows it is poisonous. So it wouldn't be in the food you eat, would it?

The answer is a little more convoluted than a simple 'no'.

## Why Use It?

Salt is mostly sodium chloride.

Decent quality salt contains many other minerals and trace elements and is generally found on the posh shelf at the supermarket. Sea salt is made by evaporating seawater. Rock salt is mined directly out of the ground.

Cheap salt, more commonly known as table salt, consists of small granules, or crystals. Production involves pumping water underground into salt deposits, a process known as hydraulic mining. The salt dissolves in the water, turning the water into brine, and this is then pumped back up to the surface. The water in the solution is evaporated, and salt crystals form.

When economies of scale are factored in, hydraulic mining is the most cost-effective way of producing salt.

It also allows purification steps to be added to the process, with the resulting salt being almost 100% sodium chloride.

If left to its own devices, table salt will absorb water and those little crystals will begin to clump together.

This isn't an ideal situation.

The solution to the problem is to add an anti-caking agent. If you look on the back of a packet of salt you will see if it contains such a thing.

Most commonly, it is listed as Sodium Hexacyanoferrate.

## What's the Problem?

The 'cyan' part of the word hexacyanoferrate refers to cyanide.

The word 'hexacyanoferrate' was invented as a marketing term, to avoid the potential for reticence from consumers if they found the word 'cyanide' listed on the back of their salt.

The correct chemical term is ferrocyanide.

The chemical structure of ferrocyanide is six cyanide molecules bound to a single iron atom.

It is considered safe because the cyanides are tightly bound to the iron, so the ferrocyanide (allegedly) doesn't release free cyanide in the body.

Another more creative name for it is "yellow prussiate of soda".

Here's a quote from **foodadditives.net**, intended to put your mind at rest...

> *Many salts of cyanide are dangerous, but the cyanide in food grade ferrocyanides is non-toxic as it is tightly bound to an iron atom and so **does not tend** to release free cyanide.*

I've highlighted 'does not tend', which makes the above statement very different from a simple, 'does not'.

**Wikipedia** has a page about sodium ferrocyanide. Here are a few quotes...

*However, like all ferrocyanide salt solutions, addition of an acid or exposure to UV light can result in the production of hydrogen cyanide gas, which is extremely toxic.*

*It is used as a stabilizer for the coating on welding rods.  In the petroleum industry, it is used for removal of mercaptans.*

*The kidneys are the organ susceptible to ferrocyanide toxicity, but according to the EFSA, ferrocyanides are of no safety concern at the levels at which they are used.*

(mercaptans produce rotten egg type smells if left in)

## Final Points

I'm always reticent to accept that low toxin levels are safe.  Sodium Hexacyanoferrrate is highly toxic in its own right, whether or not it releases cyanide gas.

The food safety argument is that it is consumed in such small amounts that you don't need to worry about it.

I'll continue to avoid it, though.

Please don't take this to mean I avoid salt. I don't place any restrictions on my salt intake, but I make sure I only use varieties that don't contain anti-caking agents.

Many websites claim various health benefits related to sea and rock salt, specifically the Himalayan pink variety of rock salt.

I'm not about to go as far as to suggest these claims are entirely valid, but as I mentioned, if you use better salt there is more probability you will get some trace elements that you'd otherwise be lacking.

I use Himalayan Pink salt because it is cheaper than sea salt, but any kind of good salt is better than eating a daily dose of cyanide.

## Further Reading

**What is Sodium Ferrocyanide (E535) in Salt and Is Cyanide in it Bad for you?**

*https://foodadditives.net/anticaking-agent/sodium-ferrocyanide/*

**Wikipedia - Sodium Ferrocyanide**

*https://en.wikipedia.org/wiki/Sodium_ferrocyanide*

**Preservation and Physical Property Roles of Sodium in Foods**

*https://www.ncbi.nlm.nih.gov/books/NBK50952/*

**How Salt Is Made**

*https://www.ncbi.nlm.nih.gov/books/NBK50952/*

**What are the 84 minerals in Himalayan pink salt?  The Complete Breakdown**

*https://www.healthmeg.com/nutrition/what-are-the-84-minerals-in-himalayan-pink-salt/*

6

# Rule 6: Don't Eat Sand

As well as being the stuff you find on a beach, sand is primarily made of silicon. This marks it out as being different to living things, which are made out of carbon.

Sand is useful when it comes to building, as it is one of the main ingredients in concrete (cement and gravel being the others)

I don't need to explain much more about what sand is (hopefully).

## Why Use It?

Powdered food ingredients tend to absorb water. Once they do so, the free-flowing powder you started with will stick together in lumps.

I've previously mentioned Microcrystalline Cellulose (wood pulp) and Sodium Hexacyanoferrate. Yet another category of anti-caking agent is based on silicon. Examples are silicon dioxide, calcium silicate, magnesium silicate, and aluminium silicate. Typically, they will absorb excess moisture and thus stop the actual ingredients, whatever they may be, from doing their lump-forming thing.

# What's the Problem?

There's no problem at all, according to various food safety organisations.

As with most of the other food additives in these rules, the amounts you are exposed to do not present any risk.

Allegedly.

Aside from anything else, sand is abrasive, so it stands to reason that the derivatives of sand are likely to have an abrasive effect on the digestive system. I don't have any science to back this up, and I don't even know if anyone has considered it.

Basic reasoning is often overlooked in the world of high science.

Looking at effects that have been studied, here's a quote from the article **Effects of Anticaking Agents and Relative Humidity on the Physical and Chemical Stability of Powdered Vitamin C...**

> *Anticaking agent type and ratio significantly affected the physical and chemical stability of vitamin C over time and over a range of RHs. No anticaking agent improved the chemical stability of the vitamin, and most caused an increase in chemical degradation even if physical stability was improved.*

So that's not too good.

Another consideration is modern production techniques. The particles of anti-caking agents are getting smaller due to industrial progress. A study looking at the effect of this, **Interactions between Food Additive Silica Nanoparticles and Food Matrices** draws the following conclusion...

> *food additive SiO2 NPs were found to interact with saccharides, proteins, fatty acids, and minerals.*

The basic finding was that the silicon dioxide reduced the bioavailability of nutrients and that more research is needed to assess toxicity.

## Final Points

It would be difficult to avoid all anti-caking agents, unless you opt for a full carnivore diet, or have time to mill all of your powdered ingredients at home.

My strategy is one of minimisation.

## Further Reading

**Wikipedia – Anticaking Agent**

*https://en.wikipedia.org/wiki/Anticaking_agent*

**Effects of Anticaking Agents and Relative Humidity on the Physical and Chemical Stability of Powdered Vitamin C**

*https://ift.onlinelibrary.wiley.com/doi/10.1111/j.1750-3841.2011.02333.x*

**Interactions between Food Additive Silica Nanoparticles and Food Matrices**

*https://www.ncbi.nlm.nih.gov/pmc/articles/PMC5461366/*

# 7

# Rule 7: Don't Eat Modified Bacterial Excrement

Starting with a vat of bacteria, you supply food to it – including warm water, sugars, carbon sources such as alcohols, acetic acid, or hydrocarbons, and nitrogen sources such as ammonia or urea. This mixture ferments, meaning the bacteria eats the stuff it is mixed with.

The 'reaction' expels waste, producing specific amino acids.

The amino acids are then isolated from the mix and modified via additional chemicals, including methanol. They are then heated and mixed before being cooled to produce crystals. These crystals are dissolved in a solvent and reacted with acetic acid, before being purified and recrystallised.

The result is **Aspartame**.

## Why Use It?

Humans are always looking for ways to have their cake and eat it. This is often in a literal way in the case of artificial sweeteners.

We want to have sweet, sugary foods, but without the sugar.

Saccharin had existed since the 1800s, and another sweetener, cyclamate, had led the creation of the diet soft drinks industry in 1953. Cyclamate was banned in the US when it was found to cause bladder cancer in rodents, leaving saccharin as the only commercial sugar substitute. In over 100 years, saccharin hadn't been able to prove itself risk-free, but by the 1970s there was huge consumer demand for sweet but low-calorie products.

Cyclamate didn't get banned everywhere, and the research that led to it being banned in the US was found to be 'flawed', opening the way for a reintroduction. However, its ban did leave saccharin as the only available sweetener for a time. Interestingly, saccharin was also shown to cause bladder cancer in rodents, but luckily that research was also found to be 'flawed'.

Whether these studies were right or wrong, they did create the opportunity for competition in the sweetener market.

A less convoluted way of saying that is to say there was huge market potential for other artificial sweeteners.

Aspartame was invented in 1965, but it didn't find its way into food and drinks until the 1980s. Since then it has become very popular with manufacturers of processed crap.

## What's the Problem?

The background information above is why I don't eat aspartame.

Even though in my mind, I don't need to go any further with this explanation, I will, as there is plenty of observational evidence to suggest it isn't the best item to be ingesting.

The **IARC** (International Agency for Research on Cancer), a division of the World Health Organisation, classifies aspartame as a Group 2B carcinogen. This means it has the potential to cause cancer.

One study, **Aspartame and Cancer - New Evidence for Causation** makes the following observation...

> *These new findings confirm that aspartame is a chemical carcinogen in rodents. They confirm the very worrisome finding that prenatal exposure to aspartame increases cancer risk in rodent offspring.*

If you apply the saccharin method of interpreting studies involving rats, then all is fine, but as with all of the chemicals I am covering, I see it as a good idea to exercise extreme caution.

The following isn't a study but is an article referencing various studies. **'What Is Aspartame?'** is well worth a read if you want an overview of the current state of research. Here's a quote...

> *Some evidence suggests consuming artificial sweeteners, like aspartame, could negatively impact the gastrointestinal microbiome, or bacteria in the gut, and promote a pro-inflammatory environment in the digestive tract.*

That statement is enough for me, notwithstanding the cancer risks. My goal when learning about all of this was to reverse the disastrous state of my digestive system, so anything that has so much as a chance of affecting it negatively is off my menu.

This is a long read, but '**Artificial Sweeteners: History and New Concepts on Inflammation**' has the following to say about aspartame...

> *The long-term consumption of aspartame has been shown to induce liver degeneration, necrosis, fibrosis, and mononuclear cell infiltration...*

It goes on to say this...

> *Prolonged aspartame consumption increases methanol and its metabolites, which are associated with oxidative stress.*

## Final Points

So that's all nice.

To conclude, I'll add that as well as my reservations about eating things that come out of chemical factories, I also don't eat aspartame because of the documented potential issues I've mentioned.

# Further Reading

**The History of Aspartame**

*https://dash.harvard.edu/bitstream/handle/1/8846759/Nill,_Ashley_-_The_History_of_Aspartame.html*

**Aspartame manufacturing process**

*https://www.madehow.com/Volume-3/Aspartame.html*

**Aspartame and cancer - new evidence for causation**

*https://pubmed.ncbi.nlm.nih.gov/33845854/*

**What Is Aspartame?**

*https://www.health.com/aspartame-7563748*

**Artificial Sweeteners: History and New Concepts on Inflammation**

*https://www.ncbi.nlm.nih.gov/pmc/articles/PMC8497813/*

8

# Rule 8: Don't Drink Disinfectant

Chlorine kills things. It doesn't particularly discriminate between different living organisms, but more of it is required to kill bigger things. Various chlorine-containing compounds can be used. This can be chlorine gas, chlorine dioxide, bleach, sodium hypochlorite, or chloramine.

With the partial exception of chloramine, they have a very distinctive smell. Chlorine gas was quite handy in trench warfare situations in World War One, as long as morals and ethics weren't factored into the equation.

## Why Use It?

Untreated water has all sorts of bugs and toxins in it. Filtration gets the bigger contaminants out. However, filters do nothing for the smaller, microscopic things like bacteria or parasites (or the eggs of parasites).

Chlorine-based disinfectants deal with most of the living things in water by killing them. As such, waterborne diseases have been eradicated in places where drinking water is treated with chlorine.

Without chlorine treatment, water would still carry diseases like Typhoid and Cholera.

So, there is a good reason to use chlorine to treat water or to disinfect surfaces.

## What's the Problem?

This isn't quite as clear-cut as with some of the other foods and additives on my list, as it is entirely reasonable to drink clean water, but there are several downsides to ingesting chlorine.

The most obvious one of these is the fact that chlorine will continue to do what it does best once inside of you, meaning it will continue to kill things. Not the whole of you, unless you directly drink some bleach. But it will kill some of the little things living inside you. The first thing in the firing line is the bacteria in your digestive system.

You will find another one of my rules telling you not to worry about your digestive flora but don't take that rule to mean it is OK to kill it all by sterilising your insides. I explain it in more depth in that rule, and my general line of reasoning is that your bacterial profile will adjust itself depending on the underlying condition of your gut, which in turn results from what you put into it. Simply wiping out whatever is in there is not going to produce good results.

According to the article **Drinking Water and Cancer**, drinking chlorinated water increases the risk of developing cancer...

*The use of chlorine for water treatment to reduce the risk of infectious disease may account for a substantial portion of the cancer risk associated with drinking water. The by-products of chlorination are associated with increased risk of bladder and rectal cancer, possibly accounting for 5000 cases of bladder cancer and 8000 cases of rectal cancer per year in the United States.*

Wikipedia has a page called **Disinfection by-product**, which, as the name suggests, explains a bit about additional by-products created as a result of adding chlorine to water. These by-products are generally toxic. Chloramine, used increasingly in modern water treatment, also produces carcinogenic by-products.

There are numerous studies and not-quite-studies, available online, with further information about the negative health effects of chlorinated water. However, basic common sense should be all that is required. As such, I'm not providing a long list of references here.

If you continually ingest something detrimental to life, it will have a negative effect. The amount doesn't matter as anything above zero is worse than none, regardless of some supposed safe level.

That being said, drinking contaminated water is worse for you in the immediate term, so there is a fine line to be navigated. This line has to do with removing the chlorine from the water before you drink it.

## Final Points

Water treated with chlorine gas, chlorine dioxide, or hypochlorite has a distinctive smell, like a swimming pool. If left to stand for some time, the chlorine will evaporate, so it will no longer be in the water.

Another problem with chlorine-treated water is that some dissolved chlorine will react with other organic compounds, producing toxic by-products.

Modern water treatment often involves chloramine instead of simple chlorine. Chloramine is chlorine bound to ammonia. It doesn't smell as much. It also doesn't evaporate out of the water in the same way as chlorine, so potentially is a bigger problem.

The options are to drink spring water or to apply considerable filtration solutions to mains water supplies.

## Further Reading

**Wikipedia - Water chlorination**

> *https://en.wikipedia.org/wiki/Water_chlorination*

**Drinking water and cancer**

> *https://www.ncbi.nlm.nih.gov/pmc/articles/PMC1518976/*

**Wikipedia - Disinfection by-product**

> *https://en.wikipedia.org/wiki/Disinfection_by-product*

# 9

# Rule 9: Don't Eat Non-Stick Cookware

Polytetrafluoroethylene (PTFE) has a long list of industrial uses. First discovered in 1938 by the DuPont chemical company, they patented it in 1941 and registered the Teflon trademark in 1945.

Known as a 'forever chemical', or a persistent organic pollutant, it is very resistant to decomposition.

If you want to read a full history of Teflon and similar chemicals, see the link to the Wikipedia page below.

## Why Use It?

It has numerous industrial applications, including but not limited to the insulation of electrical wires, the manufacture of bearings and gears, and as a coating in pipes to improve the flow of liquids (such as in brake pipes). It is also used to seal mechanical joints and is common in waterproof clothing.

However, the best-known use of Teflon is in non-stick cookware which is why it is relevant here.

I'm hoping that I don't need to explain any more about this, as I'm not looking to fill this book up with fluff. If you have non-stick cookware then it is most likely coated in Teflon.

It is allegedly safe to use in cooking as it can withstand high temperatures without decomposing or melting, so in theory it will not be affected by typical kitchen applications.

However, it starts to decompose at 250 degrees centigrade (Celsius). That isn't far above standard cooking temperatures which can reach 230 degrees.

## What's the Problem?

I'll answer this with another question.

Why do non-stick pans lose their non-stickiness over time?

It is because the non-stick coating slowly comes off. This is not necessarily because of the heat it is subjected to when heated, or the detergent it is washed with. It probably has more to do with the abrasive action of pushing food around when cooking it. It will also be due to scrubbing while washing pans and baking trays.

If bits of the coating are coming off then those bits are ending up somewhere. Some of them will go down the sink with the dishwater.

Some will mix in with your food.

According to the world of high science, only Teflon manufactured before 2013 poses any risk. It was manufactured with a chemical called Perfluorooctanoic acid (PFOA), which is carcinogenic.

If you have seen the film *Dark Waters*, it was about the PFOA used in the manufacturing process, rather than Teflon itself. If you haven't seen it, it is worth watching.

Instead of using PFOA, the manufacturing process now uses a chemical called GenX, which has been shown to carry similar risks, according to the Wikipedia page about Teflon...

> *As a result of the lawsuits concerning the PFOA class-action lawsuit, DuPont began to use GenX, a similarly fluorinated compound, as a replacement for perfluorooctanoic acid in the manufacture of fluoropolymers, such as Teflon-brand PTFE. However, in lab tests on rats, GenX has been shown to cause many of the same health problems as PFOA.*

So that's not good.

Regardless of the manufacturing processes, there is still no way it is healthy to have bits of the finished product floating around inside you.

Aside from the issues around standard usage, it is easy to burn a Teflon-coated pan. Above 250 degrees the Teflon breaks down, releasing toxic fumes. If inhaled these fumes cause Polymer Fume Fever, also known as Teflon Flu. That also isn't good.

## Final Points

There is no need to use non-stick cookware.

Cast iron or stainless steel is much less likely to be toxic. Cast iron can be seasoned relatively easily by baking some fat in the pan, after which it has its very own non-stick properties. There are also ceramic non-stick options if you don't want to use cast iron.

As with many of my rules, if a chemical-based product isn't necessary then avoidance is easier than performing an in-depth investigation.

That way I don't have to worry about the latest research or the safety data.

## Further Reading

**Wikipedia – Polytetrafluoroethylene**

*https://en.wikipedia.org/wiki/Polytetrafluoroethylene*

**Wikipedia – Dark Waters (2019 film)**

*https://en.wikipedia.org/wiki/Dark_Waters_(2019_film)*

**Fumes from Burning Plastic, Welding, and "Teflon Flu"**
*https://www.poison.org/articles/fumes-from-burning-plastic-welding-and-teflon-flu-223*

# 10

# Rule 10: Don't Eat Chlorinated Sugar

The sugar company, Tate and Lyle, was looking for ways of turning their main product into other chemicals. One of the compounds they came up with was a disaccharide (two sugar molecules joined together) composed of 1,6-dichloro-1,6-dideoxyfructose and 4-chloro-4-deoxygalactose. It turned out to be incredibly sweet.

The full chemical name is as follows...

1,6-dichloro-1,6-dideoxy-$\beta$-$D$-fructofuranosyl-4-chloro-4-deoxy-$\alpha$-$D$-galactopyranoside.

There would have been problems if anyone had tried to market a product with a name like that, so it became known as **sucralose**.

## Why Use It?

The same reasons apply to all sugar alternatives - sweetness without the sugar.

Perceptually, sucralose doesn't seem as artificial as other sweeteners such as saccharin, aspartame, and acesulfame-K. It is made out of sugar and was invented by a sugar company.

It is 600 times as sweet as sugar so a little goes a long way (I'm not sure how such things are measured, by the way). Because of this, bulking agents such as maltodextrin are often added to it. I've mentioned my thoughts about maltodextrin in another one of these rules.

## What's the Problem?

I always try to be fair and unbiased when building my understanding of things, so being honest, I'll admit that it was more difficult to find the red flags associated with sucralose, compared to its competitors.

The biggest immediate issue was the use of fillers in commercial preparations.

Unlike the less natural alternatives like saccharin, aspartame, and acesulfame-K, it doesn't have question marks surrounding whether it is carcinogenic, so that's good.

Here are a few snippets of what Wikipedia has to say about sucralose...

*during storage at elevated temperatures (38 °C, 100 °F), sucralose may break down, releasing carbon dioxide, carbon monoxide and minor amounts of hydrogen chloride.*

*There is no evidence of an effect of sucralose on long-term weight lossor body mass index, with cohort studies showing a minor effect on weight gain and heart disease risks.*

*measurements by the Swedish Environmental Research Institute have shown sewage treatment has little effect on sucralose, which is present in wastewater effluents ... warns a continuous increase in levels may occur if the compound is only slowly degraded in nature.*

Admittedly, that could be worse, but it could also be better.

A study named **Sucralose, A Synthetic Organochlorine Sweetener: Overview of Biological Issues** is a more forthcoming in presenting some possible dangers. Here are a few highlights...

*In rats, sucralose alters the microbial composition in the gastroin-testinal tract (GIT)*

*An overall reduction of the existing microflora was found ($\geq 50\%$) at sucralose doses that were lower than the human ADI. Beneficial bacteria including lactobacilli and bifidobacteria were dispro-portionately affected compared to pathogenic bacteria including enterobacteria. Further, the reduction in fecal microflora was not fully reversible even 3 mo after cessation of sucralose.*

*...found that sucralose induced DNA damage in mouse GIT(gastro-intestinal tract)*

*raises the possibility that sucralose may impact the stability of the entire bacterial ecosystem in the GIT because Bacteroidesplay a critical role in the stability and resilience of gut colonization*

*Reductions and imbalances in the composition of intestinal bacte-ria play a role in numerous medical conditions, including allergies, gastric cancer, Crohn's disease, obesity, and inflammatory bowel disease (IBD)[... ... ...] recently proposed that inhibition of intestinal microflora by sucralose is a causative factor in IBD based on epidemiological trends*

*"caution should be exercised in the use of sucralose as a sweetening agent during baking of food products containing glycerol and or lipids due to the potential formation of toxic chloropropanols."*

So it turns out there are several possible issues surrounding sucralose and digestive health.

## Final Points

In keeping with the general theme of artificial sweeteners, sucralose is implicated in upsetting the bacterial balance of the digestive system.
I don't think I'll be eating it anytime soon.

## Further Reading

**Wikipedia – Sucralose**

*https://en.wikipedia.org/wiki/Sucralose*

**Sucralose, A Synthetic Organochlorine Sweetener: Overview of Biological Issues**

*https://www.ncbi.nlm.nih.gov/pmc/articles/PMC3856475/*

# 11

# Rule 11: Don't Eat Soluble Fibre

Carbohydrate is one of the major food groups. The name refers to the carbon, hydrogen, and oxygen it is made of.

There are various ways of classifying carbohydrates into subgroups, but for this rule, the most useful way is to say they can be sugars, starches, or indigestible.

The different types of carbohydrates have technical-sounding names.

Simple sugars are called monosaccharides. Glucose or fructose are most common, and these can be absorbed into the body immediately.

Disaccharides such as sucrose and lactose are two sugar molecules joined together. They are broken down into monosaccharides before being absorbed, via the action of enzymes and water. This is why some people have a lactose intolerance, due to a lack of the enzymes required to break lactose down.

Starches are polysaccharides, meaning they are long chains of simple sugars, but the digestive system can break these down into glucose and absorb them as simple sugars.

The digestive system cannot break down certain other polysaccharides. Along with another carbohydrate group called oligosaccharides, which also cannot be broken down, these indigestible carbohydrates are known as soluble fibre.

## Why Use It?

As far as I understand it, soluble fibre exists naturally in all fruits and vegetables – some of these have much higher concentrations than others. A quick internet search will give you a list of foods with high levels. Beans, sprouts, broccoli, figs, avocados, and a range of nuts and seeds top the list.

Soluble fibre is considered beneficial to health. The only information you will get from the internet, medical people, and health and well-being experts, is to eat as much of these kinds of things as you can. If you meet your daily quota of soluble fibre then you will be healthy forever, and blah, blah, blah.

Soluble fibres, as the name suggests, are soluble in water. Dissolved, they form a gloopy, gelatinous mixture, resembling wallpaper paste.

This slows down the digestive process, keeping the stomach full for longer. In turn, this helps to prevent you from stuffing your face all day long and becoming fat.

There are also claims that it is a 'prebiotic', meaning it feeds the good bacteria in your gut, further enhancing the life-affirming nature of soluble fibre.

Things get a bit more difficult here – while companies selling prebiotics market this information as factual, real evidence for the benefits of feeding your bacteria is more difficult to find.

## What's the Problem?

If you have a healthy, intact digestive system then there is probably no downside to eating soluble fibre, except perhaps, if you consume too much and end up farting all day long – which can be considered a bit of a problem in social settings.

However, if you have inflammatory bowel disease, soluble fibres are not your friend, regardless of whatever the experts might tell you about the benefits of eating fruits and vegetables.

A study published in 2024 shows that inulin, a common type of soluble fibre, can promote intestinal inflammation.

The study is behind a paywall, but the abstract can be freely viewed.

An article explaining the details of the study, **Common type of fiber may trigger bowel inflammation**, says the following...

> *Inulin, a type of fiber found in certain plant–based foods and fiber supplements, causes inflammation in the gut and exacerbates inflammatory bowel disease...*

My understanding for soluble fibre being a problem is much simpler than any full scientific explanation. Here goes...

> In places where you have ulcers and inflammation, you don't have the protective layers of the digestive system to keep irritants away from your cells and bloodstream. Indigestible bits will reach areas they shouldn't, leading to problems not experienced by regular, healthy individuals.

There isn't much research on this subject, but direct experience tells me what I need to know.

# Final Points

I avoid soluble fibre as much as possible. This goes against all the advice I have ever received on the subject (it means not eating fruit or vegetables).

I don't worry too much about little bits and pieces of it in my food – it would be highly restrictive to remove all soluble fibre all of the time.

However, I do minimise it.

The FODMAP diet agrees with me to an extent. It is more focused on Irritable Bowel Syndrome rather than full-blown Inflammatory Bowel Disease, but my position on this is that if you have bowel disease then you can also tick all of the boxes for IBS.

Note: If you decide to follow this rule, then see my rule about Vitamin C. Then be sure to apply that one.

# Further Reading

**Dietary fiber is a critical determinant of pathologic ILC2 responses and intestinal inflammation**

*https://rupress.org/jem/article-abstract/221/5/e20232148/2766 41/Dietary-fiber-is-a-critical-determinant-of*

**Common type of fiber may trigger bowel inflammation**

*https://news.cornell.edu/stories/2024/05/common-type-fiber- may-trigger-bowel-inflammation*

# 12

# Rule 12: Don't Eat Gluten

Gluten is usually perceived as the protein found in wheat, barley, rye, and some oat varieties. The reality is a bit more complicated though – it refers to the elastic network the actual proteins form. In wheat, there are classes of proteins called gliadin and glutenin. Each of these encompasses groups of similar protein molecules.

These protein molecules can stick together to form the molecular network known as gluten, giving bread its characteristic texture.

Barley, rye, and oats have different protein molecules - hordein in barley, secalins in rye, and avenins in oat. These are also commonly referred to as gluten.

All of these grains belong to a family of grasses known as Triticeae, or wheatgrasses, and that is the common link.

## Why Use It?

Gluten makes bread possible. Its elasticity retains the air bubbles that are produced when yeast is added. This gives dough the ability to rise and gives the final product its chewy texture. Wheat contains the best gluten-forming proteins so most bread is wheat-based.

Kneading is required to give bread its characteristic texture, as the process encourages the gluten-forming proteins to bind together. However, the same proteins are still present in products that are not kneaded.

These proteins give pasta its unique texture and are present in pastries and other bakery items.

This type of food provides staple diets throughout the world.


## What's the Problem?

Some people don't do well with gluten-containing food. Estimates suggest that between 1% and 2% of the population have Celiac Disease, where gluten causes severe damage to the small intestine, triggering an immune response that can also affect other organs in the body.

A much higher percentage, roughly between 6% and 10% of people, have gluten intolerance. This is not as obvious as full-on Celiac Disease but can lead to chronic and often undiagnosed ill health. Since it can affect other organs but not always cause direct digestive symptoms, linking gluten with the problem can be difficult. It can also be difficult for a medical professional to diagnose it accurately.

Conditions that might have gluten at their root include dermatitis, fibromyalgia, a wide range of neurological disorders, and even diabetes.

It has been suggested that gluten causes an inflammatory response in all people – the study **'Is gliadin really safe for non-coeliac individuals?'** has the following to say...

> *The data obtained in this pilot study support the hypothesis that gluten elicits its harmful effect, throughout an IL15 innate immune response, on all the individuals*

It claims that gluten-containing foods are toxic to anyone, but the way the body responds to that toxicity is what defines whether someone is intolerant or allergic.

Another paper, **The opioid effects of gluten exorphins: asymptomatic celiac disease**, discusses how gluten proteins break down into morphine-like substances during digestion. Here is a quote from the conclusion...

> *The incomplete breakdown of the gluten protein, resulting in the presence of gliadin peptides with opioid effects, makes it plausible to suggest that the opioid effects of gluten exorphins could be responsible for the absence of classical gastrointestinal symptoms of individuals suffering from gluten-intake-associated diseases.*

The overall theme here is to suggest that because the proteins are susceptible to only being partially digested into substances resembling morphine (gluten exorphins), the painkilling effect of these exorphins masks the damage being done by the same gluten molecules.

It doesn't mention whether or not there is any possibility for opioid addiction to develop, but common sense would seem to indicate this is a definite possibility. If the case, it would go some way towards explaining why many people continue to stuff their faces with bakery goods, even when they are overweight.

## Final Points

The 'gluten' component in oats does not have the same toxic effect as the other grains, making oats less of a problem (allegedly).

One area that is of particular note at present is the fake meat industry. Many fake meat products use gluten proteins to give the foods a meat-like texture but at much higher concentrations than traditional breads and bakery products.

If you have any form of digestive disease, then gluten can be a good starting point when it comes to finding what the cause is. It might not be implicated, but it is relatively easy to find out – simply stop eating gluten for a while. However, while easy in principle, it can be a difficult goal to achieve, as gluten finds its way into a huge range of food products.

If you remove gluten from your diet, it is natural to find a way of replacing it. The food manufacturing industry offers gluten-free products to meet the demand, but be very careful when looking into such products. Gluten has unique properties, and foods alleging to offer something similar tend to be loaded with the kinds of ingredients you will find in many of the other rules in this book.

## Further Reading

**Wikipedia – Gluten**

*https://en.wikipedia.org/wiki/Gluten*

**Wikipedia – Triticeae**

*https://en.wikipedia.org/wiki/Triticeae*

**Is gliadin really safe for non-coeliac individuals? Production of inter-leukin 15 in biopsy culture from non-coeliac individuals challenged with gliadin peptides**

*https://www.ncbi.nlm.nih.gov/pmc/articles/PMC1954879/*

**The opioid effects of gluten exorphins: asymptomatic celiac disease**

*https://www.ncbi.nlm.nih.gov/pmc/articles/PMC5025969/*

# 13

# Rule 13: Don't Eat The Produce Of A Chemical Factory

Continuing from my other sweetener rules, it makes sense to maintain the general principle of not eating artificial chemicals. If you thought aspartame was the result of the chemistry set from hell, then hold your horses – the next sweetener under scrutiny makes it look like an example of pristine organic farming.

Here's a scrumptious little recipe...

*1) You get some acetic acid and heat it. This produces a gas called ketene.*

*2) As it cools down, ketene turns to a liquid called diketene.*

*3) Next, add some formaldehyde to the diketene. The reaction produces diacetone alcohol. (if you haven't got any formaldehyde on hand, you can make it by oxidising some methanol, or you can borrow some from your local embalmer)*

*4) Add in some nitric acid to turn the diacetone alcohol into acetoacetic acid*

*5) Add some methoxyethylamine, and you will get4,4-dimethyli midazolidinone.*

(The chemical names are getting big at this point, so don't worry if it all sounds a bit space age)

*6) After this, you chlorinate and sulfonate the 4,4-dimethylim idazolidinone to turn it into 6-chloro-1,2,3-oxathiazin-4(3H)- one-2,2-dioxide. This involves chlorine gas and sulphur trioxide. These are both highly toxic, so you might want to open a window before proceeding.*

*7) You add a splash of potassium hydroxide to the 6-chloro-1,2,3- oxathiazin-4(3H)-one-2,2-dioxide, being very careful not to get any on your hands or in your eyes as it is highly corrosive.*

The result of this process is **Acesulfame-K** (the K is the chemical symbol for potassium)

It was first discovered in 1967 but didn't make its way into food until the late 1980s.

## Why Use It?

The reasons are the same as for all artificial sweeteners.

People want sweet food without calories.

Chemical manufacturers want markets for their products. Perhaps more importantly, they want products they can patent.

Hence chemists work in laboratories all day long, inventing new chemicals.

I'm the first to admit that I am not a chemist. I am also not a food scientist. However, I don't need to be either to know that the above manufacturing process is not a food recipe.

As with all artificial sweeteners, the food standards people classify it as generally safe.

Acesulfame-K has some advantages over aspartame in terms of food manufacturing. It maintains stability at higher temperatures, making it suitable for baked goods.

However, following the initial sweet taste, it leaves a bitter aftertaste (probably something to do with all those chemicals), so it's usually combined with other sweeteners.


## What's the Problem?

Acesulfame-K doesn't break down to anything during digestion but is absorbed into the body. It (allegedly) performs no function once in the body, but the body is tasked with eliminating it, via the kidneys.

As with all artificial sweeteners, the food standards people classify it as generally safe. However...

The study, **The artificial sweetener acesulfame potassium affects the gut microbiome and body weight gain in CD-1 mice** isn't quite as confident regarding the overall safety.

Here are a few quotes from this study...

*Ace-K increased the body weight gain of male but not female mice.*

*These data suggest that perturbation of the gut microbiome by Ace-K enriched the LPS synthesis-related genes, which might increase the risk of chronic inflammation in the host.*

*Ace-K may also increase the risk of developing chronic inflammation by disrupting gut bacteria and associated functional pathways.*

*[...] could induce colitis in mice.*

*Collectively, our data evidence that Ace-K consumption can lead to adverse effects in the gut microbiome of mice.*

## Final Points

All of the above is why I don't eat acesulfame-K. I think I'll be sticking with my avoidance of it. There is a common thread throughout all studies on artificial sweeteners. They are all implicated, in some way, with disturbing the digestive biome.

I'll probably mention this more than once in these rules, but I don't think alterations in the digestive environment are the primary cause of its degeneration towards disease. However, I believe those changes are good indicators of the result of damage.

# Further Reading

**How Acesulfame Potassium is Made!  Discover the Manufacturing Process and Raw Materials Behind this Popular Sweetener**

*https://easybuyingredients.com/blog/how-acesulfame-potassium-is-made-discover-the-manufacturing-process-and-raw-materials-behind-this-popular-sweetener/*

**The artificial sweetener acesulfame potassium affects the gut microbiome and body weight gain in CD-1 mice**

*https://www.ncbi.nlm.nih.gov/pmc/articles/PMC5464538/*

# 14

# Rule 14: Don't Eat Seed Oil

First, in terms of food and cooking, oils tend to be liquid and fats tend to be solid at room temperature, which isn't entirely relevant to this rule but is useful to know. However, this key difference would seem to imply that coconut oil should be called coconut fat, but it isn't. Luckily, that also isn't relevant here.

Fats and oils come from various sources, and the ones I am talking about in this rule are extracted from the seeds of plants. Examples are rapeseed (or canola), sunflower, soybean, flaxseed (or linseed), grapeseed, sesame, cottonseed, and safflower.

The process of extracting oil from seeds is somewhat extensive.

It starts with growing plants and harvesting the seeds. These are cleaned before having their outer shells removed. The kernels are then pressed into a cake. This cake has a solvent added to liberate the oil, the solvent is evaporated off, and the oil is then bleached and deodorised. The result is a shelf-stable oil.

## Why Use It?

There are a couple of arguments in favour of using seed oils.

The first has to do with economies of scale. If you have a decent amount of farmland, a great big factory, and can implement a long distribution chain, then you can produce vast quantities of cooking oil relatively cheaply.

The second is related to alleged health benefits.

Since the 1970s, seed oils, also known as vegetable oils, have been the subject of one of the most successful marketing/PR campaigns ever.

Much of the world adopted industrially produced seed oils without question, accepting as fact claims they were the healthy option.

The liquid nature of these oils presents a slight problem in cases where solid fats produce better results. However, the industry found a solution to that issue long ago - hydrogenation. When oils are fully hydrogenated they become a hard, waxy solid. Partial hydrogenation yields a softer, more pliable product, but has the downside of introducing trans-fats into the diet (these are known to cause heart disease).

## What's the Problem?

The manufacture of seed oils is industrially intensive. This means they are, by definition, a processed food.

Large-scale production is required to make seed oils economically viable. This doesn't necessarily have any direct influence on digestive health. However, it is always good to maintain some scepticism regarding big companies and how they present their products to consumers. Science is not immune to corporate requirements.

For the supposed health benefits or otherwise, arguments for and against seed oils are plentiful (more plentiful in favour of, but that must be understood in the context of the businesses behind the arguments).

Mostly, they are presented as the healthy option, whereas saturated fats are generally seen as unhealthy, artery-clogging substances. The original arguments against fat, particularly saturated fat, originated from research by Ancel Keys in the 1960s (the **Seven Countries Study**). The findings are still disputed today, but the idea has taken root across society. Major issues with the research include cherry-picking of the countries, no separation of trans-fats (which were used extensively at that time), and no consideration of similar correlations that could be drawn from sugar intake. However, the modern food industry has built itself around the idea that vegetable oils are better and this direction isn't about to change.

I'm not going any further with the claims of health benefits or otherwise. My intention with this book is to offer you a set of simple rules for digestive health, and an analysis of the current state of research would introduce considerable complexity into this chapter.

Keeping things straightforward, I avoid seed oils because I feel much better when I avoid them.

I suffer much less indigestion if I stick to more natural fats such as lard, butter, and coconut oil.

My cholesterol levels are fine, by the way.

## Final Points

The subject of fats and oils is extensive, so a complete discussion is beyond the scope of this book, but the classification of fats has to do with the bonds between carbon atoms in the molecule. Saturated fats contain only single bonds between carbon atoms, whereas unsaturated fats contain double bonds. Monounsaturated fats have a single double bond and polyunsaturated ones have two or more double bonds.

In chemical terms, a carbon chain with double bonds is less stable than one with single bonds as there is space for other atoms and molecules to attach themselves. Saturated fats are therefore more stable. Polyunsaturated fats are the least stable, as there are multiple points on the fat molecule for other chemicals to bind to. Omega-3 and Omega-6 oils are examples of polyunsaturated fats.

Polyunsaturated fats don't respond well to heating, particularly if reheated multiple times. The 'healthy' omega oils turn into trans-fats when heated, and even mainstream sources agree that trans-fats are particularly bad. It raises questions about the production methods of seed oils, where heating is part of the process. It also raises questions about the use of such oils for cooking.

Trans fats are commonly found in processed foods and the oils used for cooking fast foods, which is enough reason to avoid such foods.

Many of the numerous scientific 'proofs' of the relative health risks or benefits, and the claims of food and nutrition experts, must be viewed through a lens of either commercial requirements or ideological stance.

So, for this subject, I mostly go with how I feel when I ingest the different types of oil or fat.

I manage much better with the old-fashioned, saturated fats for my cooking. I don't eat processed food that much and mostly never eat fast food, so I don't come across trans fats in my day-to-day life.

One other point – cold pressed oils are marketed as the high-end offering of the seed oil industry. The production of them skips the solvent-based extraction phase. However, they are still bleached and deodorised.

# Further Reading

## Seven Countries Study

*https://en.wikipedia.org/wiki/Seven_Countries_Study*

## Wikipedia: Trans fat

*https://en.wikipedia.org/wiki/Trans_fat*

## Processing Edible Oils

*https://extension.psu.edu/processing-edible-oils*

15

# Rule 15: Don't Rely on Pills and Potions

Pharmaceutical medicines are big business.

If something is wrong with you, you go to the doctor who will prescribe medication to fix whatever is wrong.

Medical drugs were originally derived from plants and some still are, so they have a heritage stretching back into the mists of time.

Then organic chemistry took over when it was discovered that oil could be turned into more than fuel and lubricants for engines.

The next great hope for pharmaceuticals was biologics – otherwise known as monoclonal antibodies.

Currently, the biotech industry has great hopes for personalised gene-based therapies.

Alternative therapies are big business as well. I've never tried them as I could never convince myself it was worth parting with my money, so I can't provide direct evidence of whether they have any effect. They do tend to be rather pricey, though.

Somewhere in the middle is the supplement industry, which is also big business.  There are all kinds of supplements, aiming to top up your nutrition and alleviate almost any problem imaginable. Some of them are probably helpful to some extent while others may not be (see my rule on Vitamin C for an example of a useful one).

Probiotics and prebiotics are a popular subset of the supplements industry and are intended to improve the bacterial environment of your digestive system. The principle of probiotics is that people with good digestive health tend to have a different bacterial profile from those with poor digestive health.

## Why Use It?

Medicines have indisputable effects on the body, hence the popularity of them.

They have measurable and proven impacts on disease.

This is a book of rules about digestive health so I'm only going to discuss medicines used to treat digestive diseases. They can reduce inflammation, stop indigestion, improve appetite, stop you from feeling sick, and fix both diarrhoea and constipation.

So, naturally, if you have a stomach-related issue, it is normal to go to your doctor for a remedy.

I have little to no experience with any form of alternative therapy, either as a patient or practitioner. Since this book is drawn from my direct experience, it wouldn't be fair to discuss these types of treatment, apart from saying they have never appealed to me.

Supplements provide the opportunity to make up for shortfalls in your nutrition, so there is some potential for these to be useful.

The thinking behind probiotics and prebiotics is that adjusting your bacterial profile will lead to better digestive health.

## What's the Problem?

The main issue with standard medicine is that the drugs don't fix the problem.

They do treat the symptoms associated with whatever the problem is. However, they don't change the roots of why that problem was there in the first place.

The medical industry isn't going to agree with me here, and as such, there are countless studies containing proof of just how effective their products are.

In the very, very short term, drugs are highly effective.

Longer term, things are not quite as clear cut.

Take, for example, anti-inflammatory steroids, commonly in the form of prednisolone. As well as stopping inflammation in its tracks, pred-nisolone increases both appetite and energy levels – all very welcome things if you have some form of IBD. However, as time goes on, negative side effects take over. Prednisolone mimics cortisol, meaning it triggers the release of glucose out of cells and into the bloodstream. It places the body into the initial stages of fight or flight. This is the cause of both the positive and negative effects – it is not genuine healing.

Monoclonal antibodies stop certain proteins from working. Ones targeted at proteins involved in inflammatory disease will help to cancel out the inflammation, leading to often dramatic improvements in health in the short term. However, proteins that cause inflammation in the digestive system have various other functions throughout the body, so monoclonal antibodies also stop these functions, which tend to be related to general immunity. This isn't a good ongoing strategy. Increased risk of serious infection along with liver, kidney, and lymph system damage are all possible.

Immunosuppressants act on bone marrow, reducing its production of white blood cells. This helps reduce inflammation. However, white blood cells also help with immunity and healing throughout the body. Additionally, red blood cell production is also reduced. Side effects can be significant and are similar to those of monoclonal antibodies.

Proton Pump Inhibitors stop your stomach from producing acid, which prevents indigestion. The only problem is you get no feedback from your digestive system, which means you cannot determine which foods agree with you and which don't. Also, a lack of acid makes protein harder to digest and reduces the absorption of minerals. PPIs are marketed as ulcer-healing drugs. I'm not going to comment beyond myself, but my ulcers never healed when I took them.

The latest discovery is in the world of genetics. A gene sequence has been identified that predisposes people to IBD, so a new world of gene therapy is just around the corner. However, it will be just as useless as the current treatments (my opinion only, by the way), and this is because all the therapies will do is prevent inflammation. Inflammation is the end product of a long set of preconditions. Gene-based therapies won't address these reasons.


Supplements do provide actual nutrients. However, working out which ones you are deficient in, if any, can present a considerable challenge. If you take supplements, check the additional ingredients - many will tick the boxes of some of my other rules. One of particular note here is microcrystalline cellulose.

With probiotics, the problem as I see it has to do with cause and effect.

Bacteria accurately indicates your digestive health so I won't argue against its relevance entirely.

It is rather more difficult to determine if a specific bacterial profile is the cause or the result of your digestive system's state of health. I don't know of any studies confirming my stance on this - which is the latter. I see a lot of circular reasoning behind many claims of the former.

My experience tells me it is possible to reverse severe bowel disease without paying any attention to the bacteria in residence.

In the past, I tried many times to improve my health with probiotics and prebiotics. None of them had any positive effects.

## Final Points

Anti-inflammatory drugs, whatever their mechanism of action, can only ever treat symptoms. Those symptoms are the result of whatever the underlying problem is.

There is an entirely valid argument for using them as a bridge – a window of opportunity for a patient to get to the bottom of what made them ill in the first place.

However, using drugs as ongoing management will only ever lead to bigger problems at a later date.

PPI medication is the devil in disguise. It can be hard to break the cycle as you can become dependent on it.

The function of bacteria is to break down dead and inorganic matter. I don't know if the bacteria is aware of this, but that is what it does in nature. In effect, it digests things that are otherwise indigestible.

Different strains of bacteria are capable of digesting different things.

Based on this fact, the bacteria you find in your digestive system can only result from what else is in your digestive system.

What is in there is mostly what you have eaten, but includes whatever might be excreted into your bowel to flush it out of your body (which is also the result of what you ate at some point).

You can eat all the beneficial bacteria you want, but if there is nothing for it to eat, it will die off. It will then be replaced by the (allegedly) bad bacteria you were seeking to eradicate by ingesting the good bacteria.

Prebiotics might have some additional impact in establishing 'good' bacteria, but see my rule on soluble fibres for reasons why you shouldn't go down this route if you have bowel disease.

If you don't eat anything toxic and nothing indigestible, you don't have to worry about your bacteria. It will sort itself out.

16

# Rule 16: Don't Eat Sugar Alcohols

Of all the available sugar alternatives, sugar alcohols are the most 'natural'. They already exist in various fruits and vegetables but at much lower concentrations than when used as sweeteners.

Common ones in foods include Sorbitol, Xylitol, Mannitol, and Erythritol. They are made via fermentation of sugars and other carbohydrates. On the surface, they should have a better safety profile than the completely artificial sweetener options.

## Why Use It?

In terms of sweetness, they are less sweet than sugar. They don't promote tooth decay, which is a positive. They have fewer calories than sugar, so, in theory, they can help people lose weight.

Sugar alcohols are often found combined with other sweeteners, partly because they aren't sweet enough on their own, but also because they help to mask bitter chemical aftertaste.

So what problem could I possibly have with this group of additives?

## What's the Problem?

A big one, unfortunately. They aren't easy to digest.

Because of this, they ferment and cause bloating. They can also cause nausea or diarrhoea. This is not a good thing to be subjecting yourself to, especially if you have inflammatory bowel disease.

Erythritol has been linked to an increased risk of heart disease.

Various sugar alcohols have been associated with a range of other health risks. While I find it a good rule of thumb to assume there's no smoke without fire, I'm not mentioning these additional claims here.

If you have ever heard of the FODMAP diet, the 'P' at the end of that name stands for Polyols, the chemical group that sugar alcohols belong to.

FODMAP is a medically recognised diet, which advises against the consumption of certain food groups in people who suffer from irritable bowel syndrome, or IBS. The general theme of the diet is that elements of food that cannot be digested ferment in the bowel and cause bloating and discomfort.

I will guarantee you that anyone with full-blown IBD (inflammatory bowel disease) will also have all the symptoms associated with IBS.

## Final Points

The fact that the intestine cannot digest them very well is all I need to know. That is why I don't eat sugar alcohols.

# Further Reading

**Wikipedia – Sugar Alcohols**

*https://en.wikipedia.org/wiki/Sugar_alcohol*

**What You Should Know About Sugar Alcohols**

*https://health.clevelandclinic.org/what-to-know-about-sugar-alcohols*

**Everything You Need to Know About the FODMAP Diet**

*https://www.healthline.com/nutrition/fodmaps-101*

# 17

# Rule 17: Don't Worry About Stuff

Stress and anxiety are emotional responses to perceived threats or challenges. While stress is a natural part of life and can sometimes be beneficial, chronic stress and anxiety can have detrimental effects on both mental and physical health.

Managing stress and anxiety is good in many ways, but not doing so could harm your digestive system. Science has created the concept of a gut-brain axis to explain this.

Stomach ulcers have long been associated with stress.

Worrying about something tends to increase the likelihood of indigestion, so there probably is some truth in such associations.

## Why Use It?

There are endless reasons for causing yourself stress and anxiety. Modern life has us chasing our tails, all day, every day, and still coming up short.

We can fear failure, rejection, and embarrassment to name but a few, and these fears fester away endlessly once initiated.

Money is always a good source of worry. If you don't have any then you can worry about finding some. On the flip side, when you do have some you can worry about losing it.

You can also worry endlessly about your health, and this can be an incredibly bountiful source of stress, especially when you have a genuine disease to be worrying about.

You can even worry about the fact you are worrying.

Our physical bodies were designed to deal with stress in the moment, such as when running away from predators or taking risks in the natural environment. This would burn up all of the associated internal chemical changes there and then, after which we would return to a relaxed state, allowing our bodies to heal.

Society doesn't always offer the means to dissipate stress and anxiety so readily though.

## What's the Problem?

There is quite a lot of research looking at connections between the brain and the digestive system. There's a link in the references to Wikipedia's page on the gut-brain axis, which you might find interesting. It goes beyond anything I need to know because I prefer to base my decisions on my lived experiences, but you might find it interesting (link below).

The NIH article, **Stress and the gut: pathophysiology, clinical conse-quences, diagnostic approach and treatment options**, is also a good starting point, having the following to say...

*Exposure to stress results in alterations of the brain-gut interac-tions ("brain-gut axis") ultimately leading to the development of a broad array of gastrointestinal disorders including inflammatory bowel disease (IBD), irritable bowel syndrome (IBS) and other functional gastrointestinal diseases, food antigen–related adverse responses, peptic ulcer and gastroesophageal reflux disease (GERD).*

Chronic stress and anxiety activate the body's fight-or-flight response, leading to the release of stress hormones like cortisol. These hormones can interfere with digestion by decreasing blood flow to the intestines, altering gut motility, and affecting the secretion of digestive enzymes.

On an experiential level (meaning not scientific), stress changes how you eat. This can go in many directions, such as overeating, starving yourself, or craving things like sugar. We all respond differently, but one common element of this response is that we do things detrimental to our overall well-being.

## Final Points

I can't tell you how to manage the stresses in your life. I can say that if you find a way of doing so, then you will be healthier.

It is especially difficult if you have an underlying disease, particularly digestion-related, because then you have something tangible to worry about. Unfortunately, though, your worrying will make it worse.

While I've provided a couple of references to this subject area, it is very well represented in scientific and medical literature if you want to know more. However, all the knowledge in the world won't stop you being stressed. The only way is by working through your problems and either accepting or resolving them.

# References

**Wikipedia: Gut–brain axis**

*https://en.wikipedia.org/wiki/Gut–brain_axis*

**Stress and the gut: pathophysiology, clinical consequences, diagnostic approach and treatment options**

*https://pubmed.ncbi.nlm.nih.gov/22314561/*

# 18

# Rule 18: Don't Eat Paint

The visual appeal of food is important, and this is where food colourings come into play. Some foods look better when they are nice and bright and white instead of shades of grey.

Titanium dioxide is as white as you can get, so it has found its way into various manufactured foods.

In terms of more industrial applications, it is also the colour in the brilliant white emulsion you use to paint your walls.

## Why Use It?

I already explained this in the 'What Is It' section above.

It makes foods look better.

It might be present in such things as sweets (candies), soups, cheeses, gravies, and pastries, to name but a few.

That is unless you live in the EU, where it has been banned as a food additive. However, the UK and the USA disagree with the position of the EU, so if you are British or American you will find Titanium Dioxide in various processed foods.

## What's the Problem?

While many websites will state categorically that it is carcinogenic or otherwise toxic, genuine evidence of serious negative health effects from titanium dioxide in food is rather more elusive.

The cancer-causing claims come from its role in the formation of lung cancer when the dust is inhaled.

One concern when it is used in food is related to size. The nature of titanium dioxide is such that much of it exists as particles small enough to fit into the nanoparticle category. Particles as small as this will pass through the intestinal barrier and are then likely to accumulate in the body.

From these two points, simple logic should be enough to indicate that an accumulation of the substance in various other organs is likely to have an equally detrimental effect as the direct inhalation of the dust does in the lungs.

Looking at direct impact on digestive health, **Titanium dioxide nanoparticles exacerbate DSS-induced colitis: role of the NLRP3 inflammasome**, has the following conclusion...

> *These findings indicate that individuals with a defective intestinal barrier function and pre-existing inflammatory condition, such as IBD, might be negatively impacted by the use of TiO2 nanoparticles.*

Another article, **The Intestinal Barrier-Shielding the Body from Nano- and Microparticles in Our Diet**, has the following to say...

> *Epithelial lesions might enable systemic translocation of nano- and microparticles into the system, eventually triggering an excessive immune response. Thus, IBD patients could be particularly vulnerable to adverse health effects caused by the ingestion*

*of synthetic particles with food. The food-additive titanium dioxide (TiO2) serves as a coloring agent in food products and is omnipresent in the Western diet. TiO2 nanoparticles exacerbate intestinal inflammation by activation of innate and adaptive immune response.*

So, whether or not it causes inflammation, if you have a digestive disease it is probably best avoided because it is likely to worsen inflammation.

## Final Points

There is no need to eat titanium dioxide.

The reason for the ban in the EU is because they were unable to determine a safe daily level, not because they found a toxic level of exposure. So the EU decided that it could not recommend any level as safe.

The UK and US take the opposing position. Since no level of toxicity is known, they have decided that it is probably safe in small amounts.

Studies do seem to indicate that it is implicated in inflammatory bowel disease.

Going back to my stance, there is no need to eat titanium dioxide.

## Further Reading

**Goodbye E171: The EU bans titanium dioxide as a food additive**

*https://ec.europa.eu/newsroom/sante/items/732079*

The Intestinal Barrier–Shielding the Body from Nano- and Microparticles in Our Diet

*https://pubmed.ncbi.nlm.nih.gov/35323666/*


**Titanium dioxide nanoparticles exacerbate DSS-induced colitis: role of the NLRP3 inflammasome**

*https://pubmed.ncbi.nlm.nih.gov/26848183/*

# 19

# Rule 19: Don't Eat Weapons of Mass Destruction

Pesticides kill pests. Generally, the intended targets are the things that eat food crops. This includes bacteria, fungi, insects, slugs & snails, and rodents. It also includes anything else that chooses to chomp on our food when it is growing. Weedkillers (known as herbicides) are also classed as pesticides.

The first pesticides were based on inorganic compounds or plant extracts. This included things like arsenic, copper, sulphur, and nicotine.

In the 1940s, synthetic compounds such as DDT were invented. This proved very profitable for the chemical industry. Lots of similar chemicals were introduced in the 1950s and 60s. DDT turned out to be incredibly toxic, and persistent (meaning it didn't degrade so built up in the food chain). DDT belongs to a group of chemicals called organochlorines.

Persistent pesticides were banned from the 1970s onwards. Allegedly less damaging chemicals such as organophosphates took over. Organophosphates are derived from phosphoric acid and are also highly effective chemical weapons. They are incredibly toxic so are slowly being replaced by newer compounds.

Carbamates are another group of pesticides and are derived from carbamic acid. They have a similar action to organophosphates so they are also highly toxic.

Neonicotinoids are derived from nicotine, and are in widespread use, with the claim that they aren't as damaging as other groups of pesticides (unless you happen to be a bee).

Pyrethrin and pyrethroid insecticides are derived from the chrysanthemum plant, and as with other pesticides, they are poisonous.

Herbicides also come under the broader definition of a pesticide. The best-known weedkiller, more commonly framed as a 'herbicide' by science types, is Glyphosate, or RoundUp.

Monsanto developed it in the 1970s, hot on the heels of their participation in the production of Agent Orange for the Vietnam War, which shows how much of a fine and upstanding company they were.

Monsanto has subsequently been bought, by Bayer. Bayer is another chemical company with a rich history of top-quality behaviour. As part of the IG Farben conglomerate in Nazi Germany, Bayer fully embraced the opportunity to perform forced medical experimentation in the concentration camps.

While all of this does indicate the ethical stance of these companies, it isn't directly relevant here.

So, back to Glyphosate, it kills weeds.

Not just weeds though – it kills most plant life.

## Why Use It?

The reasons for using pesticides are fairly obvious. We want our food to feed us, not the array of other lifeforms that wish to eat it first.

If you have ever grown any fruits or vegetables at home it is disappointing to watch your hard work devoured by pests.

So, the arguments in favour of pesticides are fairly obvious.

With herbicides, if you invent strains of agricultural plants resistant to Roundup, you can spray your fields, killing everything except the crop you want to grow. These plants are known as Roundup-Ready and are central to industrial-style agriculture.

The main argument in favour of Roundup is that it enables farms to produce enough food to meet the demands of the population.

A more accurate explanation might be that it enables centralised production, which is the lynchpin of the modern food system.

With pesticides and weedkillers, commercial crops can be grown at scale without having to worry as much about loss.

## What's the Problem?

The basic problem is that pesticides are designed to kill things, and people are not immune to this inherent feature.

If crops are treated with pesticides, then there will be residue amounts of those chemicals in the food that makes its way to your dinner table.

The food industry and the government of whatever country you live in will tell you that all is fine, and you don't have to worry about the minuscule amount of residue in your food.

If you want to believe that, then it is fine by me.

But I can't see how any amount of toxicity is good.

As well as being poisonous to plant life, weedkiller isn't too good for insects, animals, and people.

The science surrounding glyphosate is extensive. There are two distinct sides to it.

On one side the companies that produce it have all the evidence they need to prove it is safe.

On the other side, independent researchers also have all the evidence they need to prove it is extremely damaging to the environment and the population exposed to it.

This is one of those areas where it is difficult to distinguish between real science (meaning genuine observation) and corporate requirements.

The following quotes from **Is the Roundup Weed Killer (Glyphosate) Bad for You?**, should illustrate why I think it is best avoided...

*In 2015, the World Health Organization (WHO) declared glyphosate as "probably carcinogenic to humans"*

*In animal studies, glyphosate has also been found to disrupt beneficial gut bacteria. What's more, harmful bacteria seemed to be highly resistant to glyphosate*

Another article, **Is Roundup Dangerous? Can Weed Killer Cause Cancer?**, provides links to historical and ongoing court cases surrounding Roundup.

## Final Points

I'm not going too far into this subject because avoiding these products is an obvious argument.

Anything that is intended to kill things is going to stress your body, and whether you can feel immediate negative effects or not is irrelevant. The bug-killing types of pesticides are often closely related to the ingredients in chemical and biological weapons.

It isn't always possible to eat organic food only due to availability and price. However, minimising pesticide exposure by choosing organic where possible will help tip the scales of your health in the right direction.

## Further Reading

**Wikipedia: Pesticide**

*https://en.wikipedia.org/wiki/Pesticide*

**Wikipedia: Organophosphate**

*https://en.wikipedia.org/wiki/Organophosphate*

**Chemically-related Groups of Active Ingredients**

*https://www.epa.gov/ingredients-used-pesticide-products/che mically-related-groups-active-ingredients*

**Wikipedia: Agent Orange**

*https://en.wikipedia.org/wiki/Agent_Orange*

**Holocaust Encyclopedia: Bayer**

*https://encyclopedia.ushmm.org/content/en/article/bayer*

**Is Roundup Dangerous? Can Weed Killer Cause Cancer?**

*https://www.consumersafety.org/news/is-roundup-dangerous/*

**Is the Roundup Weed Killer (Glyphosate) Bad for You?**

*https://www.healthline.com/nutrition/roundup-glyphosate-and-health*

20

# Rule 20: Don't Go Without Vitamin C

***Note: If you are following my 'Don't Eat Soluble Fibre' rule, it is a good idea to follow this rule as well.***

Vitamin C, or Ascorbic Acid, is something we have to get from our diet. Unlike most animals, people can't synthesise their supply internally.

The complete molecule of Ascorbic Acid isn't required though – just the ascorbate part of it.

## Why Use It?

It stops you from developing scurvy. Scurvy is a disease where the body's cells lose their cohesion. It enjoyed considerable popularity a few hundred years ago, particularly in extended sea voyage settings. Scurvy is often perceived as a skin disease since the first visible signs of it appear on the skin, but it can also affect any organ in the body.

Vitamin C is a powerful antioxidant, meaning it helps eliminate toxicity from the body.

It is also essential to the formation of collagen. Collagen is required to heal wounds and repair tissue (hence the link between lacking vitamin C and scurvy).

## What's The Problem?

In general, most people get Vitamin C through diet alone. It is questionable whether everyone is getting enough, but most people get plenty to avoid visible signs of scurvy.

However, not developing a severe deficiency isn't necessarily the best measure of whether you are getting the optimum amount of Vitamin C.

I mentioned this at the top of this rule, but it is important, so I'll repeat it. If you are avoiding soluble fibres you need to ensure you are getting enough Vitamin C. If you are either avoiding or minimising your fruit and vegetable intake, it is a good idea to supplement, as most Vitamin C comes from this food group.

Even if you follow a traditional diet (one that includes fruit and veg), there is no harm in topping up your Vitamin C intake.

## Final Points

This rule is really simple ... Make sure you are getting enough Vitamin C.

It is more gentle on your stomach in the buffered form – usually Sodium Ascorbate.

L-ascorbate is the form you need. Most Vitamin C, whether ascorbic acid or sodium ascorbate, is a mix of L-ascorbate and D-ascorbate. It is better to buy only L-ascorbate, as D-ascorbate isn't absorbed by the body. If it doesn't specify L-ascorbate on the label, then it is a mixture of L and D. However, this usually isn't an option for buffered Vitamin C.

You can make buffered Vitamin C by mixing Ascorbic Acid with sodium Bicarbonate (baking soda).

I'm not going to provide any evidence to back up my next statement, but it is worth considering...

> *It is possible that better outcomes might result if 'inflammatory bowel disease' was renamed as 'intestinal scurvy'.*

I take a lot more Vitamin C than the recommended daily dose (as many small doses throughout the day), and I seem fine with it.

Final, final point – There is a bowel tolerance factor when you take high dose Vitamin C. Be aware of this, and learn what your limit is before taking a high dose then going out anywhere.

## Further Reading

**Encyclopedia Britannica: vitamin C**

*https://www.britannica.com/science/vitamin-C*

# 21

# Rule 21: Don't Eat Plastic

As I write this, microplastics are beginning to trend in research into health and pollution. I'm the first to admit I could do more to avoid plastic.

## Why Use It?

It is incredibly convenient for food and drink packaging and has endless industrial uses.

Arguably, modern society could not function without plastic. Food distribution chains rely on it to maintain freshness and cleanliness. One way plastic finds its way into food is for pieces of the packaging to break off. Another is for chemicals in the plastic to leach out into the food (although that is probably better described as chemical contamination rather than microplastic particles).

Technology and consumer items are often dependent on plastics for manufacturing. The result is that a lot of plastic gets discarded. It finds its way into our food sources, so we end up eating it.

## What's The Problem?

Most types of plastic don't biodegrade easily. Instead, they break down into smaller pieces of plastic and continue to do this until the pieces are microscopic. These particles then proceed to get everywhere.

They are found all over the natural world, and in almost every food chain. This includes human food.

There is a correlation between inflammatory bowel disease and microplastics. The article, '**IBD and microplastics: Is there a link?**' explains this more. Here's a quote from it...

> *In a new small-scale study, researchers have found an association between inflammatory bowel disease (IBD) and greater amounts of microplastics in stool. The findings appear in the journal Environmental Science & Technology.*

The article references the study **Analysis of Microplastics in Human Feces Reveals a Correlation between Fecal Microplastics and Inflammatory Bowel Disease Status** (link below). The full study is behind a paywall, but the abstract can be freely viewed.

## Final Points

This set of rules isn't a scientific analysis. It is more based on common sense, and there is no reasonable argument for plastics being good for us.

As with several of my other rules, minimising exposure is the only option here.

It is a good idea to avoid food packaged in plastic, as far as possible.

Science is only now beginning to look seriously into plastics and health, so much remains to be discovered about how bad they could be.

## Further Reading

**IBD and microplastics: Is there a link?**

*https://www.medicalnewstoday.com/articles/ibd-and-micropl astics-is-there-a-link*

**Analysis of Microplastics in Human Feces Reveals a Correlation between Fecal Microplastics and Inflammatory Bowel Disease Status**

*https://pubs.acs.org/doi/10.1021/acs.est.1c03924*

# 22

# Conclusion

Depending on your current dietary choices, these might seem a hefty set of rules.

Furthermore, depending on your current state of health, particularly your digestive health, they might not all be applicable.

I think everyone should seek to minimise the amount of artificial ingredients they are ingesting. It is difficult to provide a reasoned argument as to why anything artificial is good for you.

I could have made many more rules for the vast number of chemical additives in modern food, so there are quite a few more I probably should have mentioned. However, artificial additives tend to travel in packs, so if you avoid the ones I have discussed you will most likely avoid most of the others.

My rule about soluble fibres only applies if you have preexisting bowel disease. Under normal circumstances, the digestive system can deal with them. Fruits and vegetables are probably fine if your gut is reasonably intact. However, one of the problems I have seen time and time again with health advice is how little attention is paid to how 'healthy' options might not have the same positive impact for those with inflammatory diseases.

Most people are fine with gluten. It would be silly to avoid something that wasn't causing you problems. However, if you do have a problem with it or have issues you can't pin down, then cutting out gluten is probably a good move. It is addictive so going without can be a challenge to begin with. The emulsifiers commonly found in bakery goods are a different matter though - there is no good argument for eating those.

You might wonder why my list didn't feature sugar. It doesn't seem to affect me negatively, regardless of the negative perceptions applied to it. If you are overweight, then you should probably reduce your sugar intake, but if you have IBD then the chances are you will not be overweight. Sugar is linked to inflammation in the minds of doctors, nutritionists, and patients, but I can't find any direct evidence of this. High-fructose corn syrups are probably best avoided though.

I decided not to mention fluoride, not because I think it is good for you, but because I couldn't find anything linking it to digestive health. However, I don't use fluoride toothpaste and filter it out of my tap water.

Much of my diet consists of everything I have always been told to avoid - meat, eggs, saturated fat, salt (never table salt though), and sugar. I am not making any claims as to the long-term consequences. I was in something of a tough spot when I decided to adopt these choices. I had very little quality of life and was struggling to make it from one day to the next.

By doing everything I'm not supposed to, I have found a new lease of life, so my judgment over whether it is worth the alleged risk is probably different to most people.

If you have IBD, whether that be Crohn's, Colitis, or some more exotic variant, then it definitely might be a good idea to apply as many of these rules as you can. They turned my life around, and while I'm not claiming they will do the same for you, it is worth a try. You will soon know whether they lead to an improvement. You will have to go all-in on them to see any positive outcome, but you will know within a few weeks.

I can't stress this too much - always be very, very careful about stopping taking prescribed medication. While I am convinced the drugs only ever result in more underlying disease they may well be the only thing keeping you alive at the moment. I am not a doctor so cannot tell you what is best here.

Whatever your decisions, it is important to enjoy what you eat. Becoming a fanatic is never a good option.

# About the Author

**Kevin Kendall** writes about diet and health, drawing on his direct experiences overcoming long-term, severe Crohn's Disease. From a working-class background in the Northeast of England, Kevin brings a grounded, relatable perspective to wellness, offering practical insights that have helped him reclaim his health.

In addition to his current focus on nutrition, he is fascinated by the psychology of belief—what makes people embrace or reject new ideas—and explores this theme in his writing.

**You can connect with me on:**

🌐 https://www.kevink2.co.uk

🐦 https://x.com/northeastheret1

# Also by Kevin Kendall

Cut through the fluff of the modern world to find genuine answers.

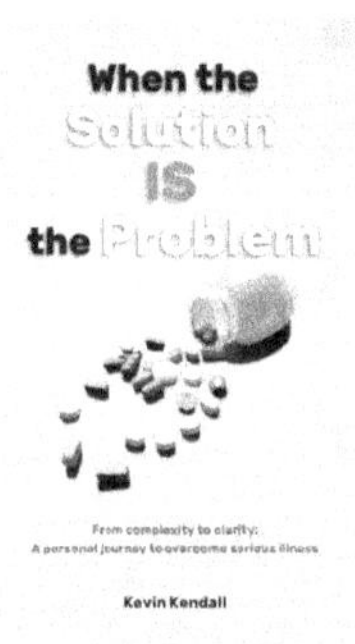


**When the Solution IS the Problem**

What if your doctor didn't know best?

Or any other expert, for that matter. Based on more than 30 years of first-hand experience, this non-fiction journey challenges conventional wisdom, showing that logic, reason, and personal responsibility can help reverse a deeply entrenched and incurable health condition.